Hydrogen peroxide (H2O2)
hydrogen and two of oxygen o
oxygen atom attached (H2O + O − H2O2). Hydrogen p---
produced in the body by certain white blood cells to fight infections as a first line of defense. Hydrogen peroxide is critical for the immune systems defense against a number of pathogens. H2O2 is an oxidative compound and is broken down by an enzyme called catalase that is stored in the cells. Catalase is also found in sprouts and in some raw vegetables. (E.G. raw potato). Add a slice of raw potato to a glass of H2O2 and this will cause bubbles of oxygen to be released. The catalase in the potato breaks down H2O2 into oxygen and water.

In 1986, I was introduced to the use of hydrogen peroxide by Walter Grotz, a retired postmaster, who had successfully treated himself for arthritis using H2O2. He had learned about using hydrogen peroxide for this purpose from Father Richard Willhelm who had studied its use for several years in the treatment of a variety of health-related conditions including arthritis.

One of the first books to document the scientific benefits of hydrogen peroxide is called ***The Therapeutical Applications of Hydrozone and Glycozone*** by chemist Charles Marchand. The eighteenth edition of this book was published in 1904. While the title of this book is about ozonated glycerin (Glycozone) and ozonated water (Hydrozone), it also contains reprints of more than 140 articles appearing in medical journals from 1888 to 1904 on the uses of peroxide of oxygen as it was originally called.

Several articles are reprinted in this book from the Journal of the American Medical Association. Some of the many diseases successfully treated with 3% hydrogen peroxide in Charles Marchand's book were - pneumonia, scarlet fever, diphtheria, whooping cough, tonsillitis, cancer of the womb, lupus, tuberculosis, gastritis, gonorrhea, gangrene, urethritis, gun shot wounds, nephritis, ear infections, sore throat, typhoid fever, yellow fever, cholera, measles, poison ivy, riggs' disease, endometritis, vaginitis, insect bites, bees stings, ringworm, emphysema, acne, hives, chilblains, piles (hemorrhoids), leucorrhoea, anthrax and periodontal disease. This was all before 1904!

We are indebted to Walter Grotz of Delano, MN, for his discovery and publication of this historical treasure that was retrieved from the Library of Congress.

Most consumers have had experience with the hydrogen peroxide that comes in a brown bottle. The 3% solution sold in pharmacies and grocery stores is stabilized with additives. It is used mainly as a mouth rinse and disinfectant or as an antiseptic for topical application. For occasional use to treat gingivitis, some dentists have recommended dipping a tooth brush in $H_2O_2$ solution and then in baking soda to brush the teeth and gums. This treatment has been used intermittently (up to 7 days consecutively) to clear out infections in the mouth and gums. It is not recommended for continuous daily use. Today, a number of brands of toothpaste on the market contain either baking soda or peroxide or both.

In his book, Hydrogen Peroxide - Medical Miracle, Dr. William Campbell Douglass M.D. writes: *"$H_2O_2$ is involved in all of life's processes. Hydrogen Peroxide is truly the wonder molecule. The cells in the body that fight infection, called granulocytes, produce $H_2O_2$ as a first line of defense against every type of invading organism - parasites, viruses, bacteria and yeast."* Sixty percent of our white blood cells consist of Neutrophils, a granulocyte that produces $H_2O_2$ to fight infections.

In presenting the positive benefits of $H_2O_2$, I have also provided information on the dangers of storing $H_2O_2$ in a refrigerator or in an unmarked bottle and the hazards of accidental ingestion of high concentrations of $H_2O_2$ and safety factors regarding the storage of hydrogen peroxide.

*Conrad LeBeau* – Feb 15th 2009

---

**Ninth Amendment, US Constitution**
*"The enumeration in the Constitution of certain rights shall not be construed to deny or disparage others retained by the people."*

Freedom of Choice in Medicine is a constitutional right retained by the people and ignored by the government. Until the Federal Government stops imposing expensive patented drugs as the first line of treatment and allows for low cost, traditional and natural medicine in the marketplace, the high cost of health care will not come down. Competition in the marketplace is the answer to more affordable and effective health care.

# Chapter I

## A bit of history

Hydrogen Peroxide was first reported by the French chemist Louis-Jacques Thenard in 1818, who named it eau oxygenee. Little is known about the use of hydrogen peroxide before the 1880's except to references in published literature of the period that it was used to treat topical wounds as a disinfectant. In the period following the Civil War, H2O2 was known as hydrogen dioxide and by 1890 was called Peroxide of Hydrogen. 3% H2O2 was labeled as 15 Volume, a reference to the volume of oxygen gas stored in the solution.

An article appeared in the New York Medical Record on October 13, 1888 about the use of peroxide of hydrogen in the treatment of Diphtheria at the Metropolitan Throat Hospital at the University of Vermont. In this report, George B Hope MD states: *"several cases of well-marked buccal diphtheria were treated with the peroxide, with the effect of confirming in the most satisfactory manner the results obtained by Dr. Bleyer* (1).

### Scarlatinal Diphtheria
by WM F Waugh M.D.

From *The Times and Register*, Philadelphia, March 7, 1891

*I desire to place upon record a case that is unique in my own experience; though my readers may, perhaps, have better results. The case was that of a child under four years of age. He had been attended by a dispensary physician during the first part of the illness; and this gentlemen, when he gave up the case, had given a gloomy prognosis, with which I heartily coincided.*

*On my first visit, I found the child's throat covered with blackish sloughs, the lips and tongue covered with fissures and ulcers, the nose discharging freely the irritating and offensive secretions of nasal diphtheria, the pain in the forehead, so that the disease had passed up the Eustachian tubes and into the frontal sinuses. Reddish spots and blotches appeared on the face and body. The stench was dreadful, the urine totally suppressed, but the few drops that were passed could not be saved for examination. The child had been delirious for some time, not being able to recognize his parents. The one good point was that his stomach retained milk fairly well.*

It has not been my good fortune to witness the recovery of many such cases. In fact, the more extended is my experience with diphtheria, the more I dread it; especially when it has become firmly established in the Schneiderian mucous membrane, and in the passage leading from the naso-pharynx.

I felt it my duty to inform the parents that death was the only result to be expected; and that they could be very thankful if their other children, six in number, should escape.

However, I gave them a bottle of Marchand's Peroxide of Hydrogen, and directed them to syringe the nostrils and wash the mouth out with a solution diluted to one-fourth employed. **This was repeated every hour, day and night.** No other treatment was employed, and whiskey was given with milk, as the only food. The child began at once to improve; the right tympanic membrane gave way, and then the solution was thrown in to the ear, and bubbled out at the nose. The urine began to be secreted more freely, and the child was pronounced out of danger one week from my first visit.

One of the other children was seized with a sore throat, enlarged tonsils and torticollis; another had a mild attack of scarlatina, but the others escaped without contracting the disease. This in itself is notable, as the children were all kept at home, in a crowded little house, with miserable sanitation.(1)

Note: What is notable about this report was the persistence of washing out the mouth and nostrils with diluted hydrogen peroxide every hour of the day and night for 7 days. No doubt, some of the $H_2O_2$ was absorbed from the mouth and sinuses into the blood and killed the virus that caused the diphtheria. This was evidently a success case of sublingual absorption of hydrogen peroxide.

## Peroxide of Hydrogen in Typhoid Fever
by F.H. Wiggin MD  From *New York Medical Record*, Nov., 28 1891

Having had good results in using Peroxide of Hydrogen locally in diphtheria and tonsillitis, and in infected wounds, it occurred to me, when a case of typhoid fever came under my care, during my summer practice, that this remedy might be beneficial, it being the most powerful non-poisonous germicide we possess.

On August 24th I was called to see Abby M-, who gave a history of having been ill for a week with fever and diarrhoea. On examination I found a characteristic case of typhoid fever and temperature of 104 and $1/2°$ F.; pulse, 130; rose spots, abdominal pain, tympanites diarrhoea, *and mild delirium. I prescribed one ounce of 15-volume Peroxide of Hydrogen to eight ounces of water, to be taken every 3 hours by the mouth. On the following day I found the patient more comfortable; temperature 103° F.; pulse 112; had had only two movements during the twenty-four hours; less delirium and less pain in the head. On the 26th had had one movement; temperature 102° F; pulse 104; less tenderness in abdomen, and pain in the head diminishing. On the 27th, temperature 100 and 1/2° F.; pulse 98, no movement; tympanites disappeared, and head, though still weak, clearer. On the 29th, temperature 99 and 1/2° F.; no movement. On the 30th, temperature normal, pulse 84; formed movement. The case went on uninterruptedly to recovery, with nothing further of interest to report. On the 9th of September I discontinued my visits, the patient being discharged, cured, though weak. (1)*

**Editor's Note: August 4, 2004.** This apparently is the first recorded case of using hydrogen peroxide orally (drinking $H2O2$ diluted with lots of water) to treat an otherwise fatal infection. In calculating the strength of one ounce of 15 Vol. (3%) $H2O2$ to 8 ounces of water, it would appear that based on experiences of the past decade that the dose was high enough to treat 2 or 3 patients simultaneously and bordered on an $H2O2$ overdose. One ounce of 3% $H2O2$ solution contained the equivalent of 40 drops of 35% $H2O2$ solution. If 5 glasses of this mixture were consumed in one day, it would have been the equivalent of 200 drops of 35% $H2O2$ in a 24 hour period and this is highly unlikely. It is more likely that the patient consumed less than the doctor prescribed, perhaps half or less of the prescribed dose. The highest amount I ever heard anyone using orally in the 1990's in a single day is 20 drops of the 35% $H2O2$ solution in a glass of water 5 times a day or 100 drops total. The patient of 1891 must have sipped on the mixture and probably consumed less than the prescribed dose.

An article appearing in ***The Lancet***, a British medical journal, on Feb. 21, 1920, titled: "Influentzal Pneumonia: The Intravenous Injection of Hydrogen Peroxide" tell of a remarkable recovery of a man in a coma near death who received a single injection of 3% hydrogen peroxide. While the patient recovered, the use of 3% $H2O2$ solution as an injection would not be used today as it is too strong and might just as likely kill the patients with a gas embolism.

Today, IV $H2O2$ is buffered and is diluted to less than a third of 1 percent and is administered very slowly to prevent a gas embolism. Physicians have received training from the International Bio-Oxidative Medicine Foundation (IBOMF) in safe procedures for administering diluted iv H2O2 solution as well as ozone injections or treating the blood with ozone.

## Different Grades of Hydrogen Peroxide solution

The controversy over grades of H2O2 solution actually started over a century ago and continues to this day. In 1892, an article by WB Dewees MD was published in the *Medical Record*, St. Joseph. MO. It is titled "Medicinal vs. Commercial Peroxide of Hydrogen. In it Dr. Dewees states:

*Like most of my brethren, I took it for granted that H2O2 was the same, so long as it was made by our leading manufacturing chemists, and consequently paid no attention as to the effects of brands....I have used three different products alike in abscesses of almost every description, ulcers, gangrene, cancer, endometritis, specific vaginitis, diphtheria etc, etc, and in each and every instance Marchand's preparation proved above all, not only the most effectual, but in every way a most satisfactory agent for arresting pus formation, and as a non-irritating antiseptic for general use."* (1)

In Marchand's book is a reference to phosphoric acid, sulfuric and hydrochloric acid being added to H2O2 as stabilizers. Marchand's H2O2 apparently added only a small amount of acetic acid and not enough to be irritating. Today it is known that hydrogen peroxide is unstable at a pH higher than 4.0. Today there is commercial grade H2O2 with stabilizers added, Food Grade H2O2 and Reagent grade – the purest form.

## Lemon Juice stabilizes H2O2 solution.

In a home experiment I had conducted with food grade quality 35% H2O2 solution, I added one tablespoon of pure lemon juice to 8 ounces of the solution. It lowered the pH to 2.5, well within the pH range for stability. A test bottle which I set near a south facing window exposed to direct sun light has not shown signs of a buildup of pressure after several days. Lemon juice appears to be one way of stabilizing H2O2 solutions at various concentration levels.

Ref: 1. *The Therapeutical Applications of Hydrozone and Glycozone*, by Charles Marchand, Chemist. 1904 - 18th edition. (Reprinted in 1989)

# Chapter II

# Case reports
# Rosenow, Willhelm and Grotz

Early in 1986, a farmer in Harmony, Minnesota told me how he used hydrogen peroxide to treat his farm animals for mastitis and other conditions. Inquiring further, the farmer directed me to another Minnesota resident, Walter Grotz, who shared his personal experiences with H2O2 with me.

Grotz told me of his introduction to H2O2 that he had first heard of four years previous when he and his wife took a Caribbean cruise. At that time, he had a painful arthritic condition. It was on this trip that he met Father Richard Willhelm of the Catholic Health Organization, who told him about H2O2 and how it helped other people with arthritis. Reportedly, Father Willhelm received his knowledge about H2O2 from Dr. Edward Carl Rosenow (1875-1966), who was associated with the Mayo Clinic and had authored numerous medical articles.

Upon returning from his vacation, Walter Grotz made a diluted solution of H2O2 from highly concentrated 35% H2O2 (Food Grade) solution and began to use daily the equivalent of 5 drops of 35% H2O2 solution in a glass of water 3 a day and gradually increased the dose to 15 drops 3 or 4 times daily after about 2 weeks.. In his own words, Walter claims: *"I first felt an improvement 16 days after starting on the peroxide program. In less than 2 months, all pain and symptoms of the arthritis were completely gone. For the past 4 years, I have been completely free of this disease."*

Walter Grotz provided the names and addresses of people with Arthritis, Lung Cancer, Colon Cancer, Emphysema, Diabetes and Multiple Sclerosis who claim to have benefited from the use of H2O2, with some reporting remissions of their illness.

H2O2, reportedly kills a wide spectrum of germs and viruses. However, to balance out this information, the author is aware of persons with some of the preceding conditions who did not recover or had more limited benefits after using H2O2 orally. The use of oral H2O2 remains controversial to this day with both supporters and detractors. In 1986 I learned the hard way not to mix hydrogen peroxide with iron containing well water and then drink it orally. A sore stomach was the result after free radical formation from this combination. Experience has shown sublingual absorption to be safer.

## H2O2 for Pneumonia

A. Anderson from Franksville, WI, told me how he got rid of pneumonia in 24 hours by drinking 3 glasses of distilled water. To each glass was added 10 drops of 35% H2O2. Al said he had suffered from pneumonia for about one week when he was persuaded to try H2O2. He said he was very skeptical that it would work, but was shortly surprised at the speed of his recovery. He said how the soreness in his lungs had disappeared and his normal breathing had been restored, all in less than 24 hours after taking the H2O2.

Note: **1/2 teaspoon of 6% H2O2 or 1/4 tsp. of 12% solution contains the equivalent of about 7 and 1/2 drops of 35% H2O2.**

## Dr. Christian Barnard

A world renowned physician, the late Dr. Christian Barnard, MD. Ph.D., took a small amount of diluted H2O2 daily for his arthritis. Dr. Barnard is the South African physician who made the world's first heart transplant operation. Writing to a person in England on March 10, 1986, Dr. Barnard wrote,

*Dear Mr. Wright;*

*Thank you for your letter of February 25, 1986. It is true I have found relief from the arthritis and I attribute this to taking hydrogen peroxide orally several times each day. I learned of this treatment from Mr. Walter Grotz and suggest that you could possibly write to him for further data regarding this treatment.*

*Best Wishes*
*Christian N Barnard, MD, Ph.D.*

## Reports of H2O2 results

In one instance, a lady with arthritis sprayed 3% H2O2 (from a Pharmacy) on her sore joints and experienced nearly complete relief from pain in only one week.

I know one man 80 years old who had both his hands swollen from arthritis and who applied Peroxy Gel to it regularly for one month. He told me the swelling went down and the pain was gone after applying it for only 30 days.

There have been several reports of people with Prostate problems, and other cases with Emphysema being helped tremendously with the use of a hydrogen peroxide gel absorbed externally. It is applied to the bottom of the feet and also over the chest area.

In Sonora, CA, the owner of a health food store says she shrunk a large tumor with adhesions using a hydrogen peroxide based gel. She claims the tumor, which was the size of a hen's egg, has shrunk to the size of a half-dollar and the pain is gone.

In Scottsdale, AZ, a registered nurse with an inoperable cancer, claims to have eliminated all pain by following a vegetarian diet and using 1/2 Tablespoon of Peroxy Gel three times a day. (She absorbed the equivalent of about 67 drops of 35% $H_2O_2$ into her skin each day). Her case is remarkable, since the Oncologist told her one year ago she would die in 3 months. He was surprised to see her in Jan, 1990 for a catscan and physical checkup. The catscan showed her blood to be normal and that the mass of tumor in the pancreas area was gone, leaving a small indentation. The doctor said; *"This is amazing."*

Another person at a National Health Federation Convention claims to have shrunk a tumor by mixing 1 part of 35% $H_2O_2$ with 5 parts of aloe vera juice and applying it directly on the tumor. Note: if 3% or 6% $H_2O_2$ solution is used, mix 1 part with an equal amount of aloe vera juice.

Reatha C. of Pomeroy, Ohio says she got rid of her rheumatoid arthritis which she had for 17 years using hydrogen peroxide externally. She wrote: "I've even gone back to square dancing which I haven't done for 10 years."

Note on hip joints: $H_2O_2$ will not provide relief when hip joints have deteriorated.

## H2O2 for stubborn Sinus and Lung Infections

In the spring of 1995 my mother, 81 years old at the time, had a sinus and lung infection with a cough that lasted more than 6 months. The use of herbal remedies and even antibiotics failed to clear the infection. Finally, in desperation, I suggested she try oral $H_2O_2$ and water. She took one teaspoon of a 6% $H_2O_2$ solution with a glass of water 4 or 5 times a day between meals for 3 days. On the 4th day, the cough and the low level infection were completely gone. No further use of $H_2O_2$ was needed. On a personal note, I once successfully used a small amount of oral $H_2O_2$ to overcome a stubborn sinus infection myself.

Note: Personally, I have found that milk, ice cream and some types of cheese promote sinus and lung infections and even rheumatoid arthritis.

## H2O2 for Pets

Mr. Grotz reports that the Bird-Man of Alcatraz used to add H2O2 to the drinking water of his pet birds, to treat them for a variety of illness. He is reported to have been very successful with the use of hydrogen peroxide.

In July, 1986, some friends of mine treated their sick cat with H2O2. The cat had ran away from home and had picked up a serious infection. The cat was so weak and ill it could barely stand up. They forced 2 tablespoons of a 1% solution of H2O2 down the cats throat. This was done by adding 2 teaspoons of 3% H2O2 to 4 teaspoons of water. Ten hours later, the cat had so improved that it had to be chased all over the house to catch it and give it another peroxide treatment. Within one week, the cat had completely recovered.

(Note: July 3, 1987. It is almost one year after the cat was treated with H2O2. It is alive and well).

## Hydrogen Peroxide for House Plants, Crops and Farms

For houseplants, add one tablespoon of 6% H2O2 to one quart of water and use as a foliar spray once a week. There have been several reports of plants growing healthier and faster with the foliar spray which I have been told increases nitrogen absorption.

Farm with EASE (Maxville, Ontario, Canada) reports that farmers are using 1 cup of 35% H2O2 in 20 gallons of water to spray 1 acre of crops and are getting noticeable results in increased growth of plants. They also report that farmers are preventing Mastitis in cattle by adding 30 ppm of H2O2 to the drinking water on a regular basis. **This is the equivalent of about 1 teaspoon of 35 % H2O2 to 13 gallons of drinking water.** For more information about the use of H2O2 for agricultural purposes, you can call them at 613-527-3060. Note: H2O2 as a foliar spray is reported to increase absorption of nitrogen.

## Skin absorption of H2O2 (in a bath tub)

A safe way to take Hydrogen Peroxide is to have it absorbed into your body through your skin. Many people remain skeptical that this method works. Consider this: Doctors use to have heart patients swallow nitroglycerin tablets for angina. Now they tape a tablet to their chest and it is directly absorbed into their bloodstream through the skin. The results are the same.

Some people who absorb large doses (30 drops or more of 35% daily) over a period of several months often notice their hair turning a shade or two lighter in color.

One way to take hydrogen peroxide externally is to add 6 pints of 6% H2O2 solution to a bath tub half full of water. If using drug store 3% H2O2 solution, an equivalent amount would be 12 pints. I know one person who had chicken pox and did this only once and then rapidly recovered.

Hydrogen Peroxide is an oxidizing bleach, that after being absorbed into the bloodstream, increases the level of O1. O1, released from H2O2, destroys germs and viruses of all kinds on contact. H2O2, broken down, becomes O1 plus water (H2O).

## Gerson Therapy and Cancer

Aug 9th, 1986: Jim LeBeau and I attended the National Health Federation convention in Chicago. At the convention, I met Charlotte Gerson, whose father, Max Gerson MD, pioneered the raw food juice method of treating cancer patients. She told of the many cases they successfully treated at her clinic in Mexico and how much more successful the results were since injecting (infusing) through a slow i.v. drip a diluted form of hydrogen peroxide in the patients' veins. Charlotte now claims to have doubled the number of cancer remissions in patients treated at her clinic. The Gerson Clinic also uses ozone as part of their protocol.

One of the most impressive parts of Charlotte Gerson's talk was when she told of how they located several of the patients Dr. Gerson had treated for terminal cancer 30 years ago and found that many of them were still alive! That is living testimony to the effectiveness of a treatment that did not merely treat the cancer, but treated the entire body. These earlier successful cancer patients did not use earlier H2O2 or ozone. Dr. Donsbach also shared his experiences using infusion of H2O2 at his clinic in Mexico with some of his patients sharing their experiences.

## Relapses of Candidiasis reported

While Dr. Donsbach reported several cases of ridding the body of systemic yeast infection with both oral and intravenous hydrogen peroxide, the author is aware of a number of cases where the abrupt ending of hydrogen peroxide therapy resulted in the reoccurrence of

Candidiasis. The relapse into systemic yeast infection is less likely to occur if the use of hydrogen peroxide is gradually tapered off over a period of 3 to 4 weeks and you then successfully implant friendly flora in the intestines. For information on how to do this, see my book on **"Natural Remedies for Intestinal Health."**

Note: Chronic candidiasis may also be associated with an underlying and active infection of Human Herpes Virus, variant A (HHV-6A) and a deficiency of selenium. The use of plant-based selenium "Phytosel" from Indian Mustard Greens or Broccoli has been very beneficial as has been Brazil Nuts. A maintenance dose is 400 mcg daily while a therapeutic dose of plant-based selenium in 400 mcg twice daily. A man made version of selenium called L-seleno methionine as well as yeast based selenium and sodium selenite have proved to be far less effective in numerous case reports than the 100% natural form. The manufactured form of L-seleno methionine has shown to have no benefits at all and is not safe to use above 400 mcg daily. Unfortunately this latter form, L-seleno methionine, a synthetic amino acid complex misidentified as a chelate, is the least expensive and most widely form sold in the United States.

Immune-base therapies (Fish Oil – DHA/EPA – 2000 mg daily Naltrexone - 3 to 4.5 mg daily, IP6, Aged garlic extract, Maitake, shiitake, transfer factor, beta glucan etc) help to prevent the return of candidiasis. Information on these therapies can be found in the book on **Immune Restoration Handbook** or at www.keephopealive.org

## i.v. use of hydrogen peroxide or ozone

On June 25th, 1986, I called Walter Grotz. He had just returned from a National Health Federation convention in California, where he and Dr. Donsbach had presented their latest findings. Mr. Grotz told me that *"Dr. Donsbach is infusing H2O2 at his clinic in Mexico."* Grotz reported that a terminal patient with prostate cancer made a complete recovery in 2 weeks, returned to his home in Minnesota. Still one has to wonder how do you determine who recovers and who has made a complete recovery? How long will this recovery last?

When I spoke with Grotz, I asked him what infusing was and he replied that infusion is an intravenous solution of a very diluted form of H2O2. Following this was a discussion of how infusion therapy worked.

While there was substantial enthusiasm for using highly diluted i.v. H2O2 solution in 1986, my opinion in 2005, is that i.v. ozone or autohemotherapy (ozonated blood) is a safer and more effective treatment than i.v. hydrogen peroxide solution. My views are based on several case reports from persons who tried both types of bio-oxidative therapies over the past several years.

## Sublingual absorption of H2O2 with Aloe Vera juice

I recommend a 2% H2O2 solution in a base of aloe vera juice and used by the drop for sublingual absorption in the mouth for the most benefits and with no known side effects. Two parts of a 6% H2O2 solution (food grade) is mixed with 4 parts of aloe vera juice to make a 2% H2O2 solution in aloe vera. For adults, 20 to 40 drops of this 2% solution are used sublingually under the tongue every 30 to 60 minutes or less often as needed. After holding for 3 minutes, drink a full glass of water to wash down what little you did not absorb. The aloe vera works better than plain water with H2O2 in helping absorb the H2O2 through the mucus membranes and into the blood vessels.

In the 1980's, the early promoters of H2O2 advised against using drugstore 3% H2O2 that contains chemical stabilizers.. **However, I have known persons who have used regular 3% H2O2 orally without any apparent side effects from the stabilizers.** *I am not aware of any harmful effects from the oral use of 3% H2O2 that only contain phosphoric acid, a common food additive.* However, having said that, some over the counter brands have caused nausea and are irritating due to unknown additional stabilizers added to the H2O2 solution *that are not listed on the label.*

Until recently, food grade hydrogen peroxide was only available in high concentration of 35% which must be diluted before using. Today, some companies are making it available in 6% or 12% solution. **Health food stores are strongly encouraged to ask their suppliers to provide them with a 6% Hydrogen Peroxide solution (Food Grade) for the public's use to eliminate the hazards of storing 35% solution in the home.** *35% H2O2 should only be sold to health care professionals.* Hydrogen peroxide should only be stored and made available in a brown bottle or solid white bottle but never a clear bottle where it can be mistaken for water.

Food grade H2O2 can be naturally stabilized by adding enough lemon juice until the pH of the solution reaches 3.0. Note: Use pure lemon juice without additives in it.

# Chapter III
# Hydrogen Peroxide and Cancer
# The scientific evidence

An article in Radiation Research magazine in 1977 by E. B Watkins and D.G. Willhoit titled "The Combined Effects of Hydrogen Peroxide and Y Radiation on the Mitotic Activity of Ehrlich Ascites Tumor Cells" discusses the enhanced effects of combining infusions of hydrogen peroxide with radiation in the treatment of cancer. On H2O2 alone, they wrote: "Hydrogen peroxide, used alone, has been shown to delay the appearance and development of the Ehrlich ascites tumor and this, consequently, increases the survival time of the host animal." They refer to another article appearing in Radiology 82, 322-324 (1964).

In October, 1965, in CANCER, published by the American Cancer Society, is an article titled "Regional Oxygenation in the Diagnosis and Management of Intra-abdominal and Retroperintoneal Neoplasms" by Drs. Arnoff, M.D., Balla, M.D., Finney, M.A., Collier, M.D., and Mallams, M.D.. They wrote: The resection of this tumor apparently was made possible by presurgical medium dose irradiation associated with regional oxygenation by the intra-arterial infusion of a solution of hydrogen peroxide into the abdominal aorta."

In CANCER magazine June, 1989, is an article titled "In-Vitro Sensitivity of Hodgkin's Disease to Hydrogen Peroxide Toxicity" by Samoszuk M.D., Rietveld M.A., Gidanian B.S., and Petersen B.S.. Interestingly enough, they wrote: "ionizing radiation readily generates quantities of hydrogen peroxide by radiolysis of tissue water." In layman's language, radiation produces small amounts of hydrogen peroxide inside cancer cells which may explain in part how the cancer cells are destroyed! There is no evidence that the oxygen in atmospheric air, O2, will destroy cancer cells. Existing scientific research indicates it takes the free radical form O1 to accomplish destruction of cancer cells. H2O2 breaks down into water (H2O) and O1. This breakdown is done by an enzyme called catalase.

In theory, if you could increase the amount of catalase at or in the cancer mass while using iv H2O2 or even oral ingestion, it should accelerate the destruction of the cancer cells. As raw potatoes are a known source of catalase, the consumption of raw potato juice a few hours before or after the use of H202 might enhance its antiviral and anticancer effects. So far, this kind of experiment has not been done and readers are advised to consult with a health care professional before attempting this experiment on their own.

The following scientific articles were retrieved from the Medical Library in Rockville, MD: "Hydrogen peroxide and irradiation of Tumors" by WD Chasin, CC Gross, CC Wang and D Miller published in Arch Otolarygol, 1967 Feb; 85(2):151-5. "Intra-arterial infusion of hydrogen peroxide in radiotherapy of malignant tumors" by G. Bianchini, G. Salgarello, T. Mennini, and G. Lorini. It was published in Radiol Med, (Torino, 1969, Mar;55(3):207-25). "Radiotherapy of tumors under conditions of regional hyperoxygenation", by G Ambesi, C Nervi, M Cortese and C Casale titled. It then refers to "Hydrogen Peroxide/Administration and dosage." It was published in Radiol Med (Torino) 1969 Mar; 55(3):193-206. "Protracted intra-arterial chemotherapy with sequential courses of antimitotics and hydrogen peroxide in the treatment of head and neck tumors." It is written by C Nervi, C Casale and M Cortese. Published in Rev Fr Etud Clin Biol 1969 Jan; 14(1):51-4. "Hydrogen Peroxide and cytolytic factor can interact synergistically in effecting cytolysis of neoplastic targets", by DO Adams, WJ Johnson, E Fiorito and CF Nathan. It was published in the Journal of Immunology, 1981 Nov; 127 (5):1973-7 It says: "Two secretory products from activated macrophages, which are thought to be involved in the lysis of tumor cells, are H2O2 and cytolytic factor.......The data suggests that H2O2 and CF can interact synergistically to produce cytolysis of neoplastic targets...".

In layman's language, this means that hydrogen peroxide and CF is produced by the body's own immune system to destroy cancer cells! Normal healthy body cells are protected from damaging effects of hydrogen peroxide by the enzyme "catalase." Cancer cells do not have this protection.

The Journal of Interferon Research, Vol 3, No 2, 1983 said in an abstract that "The results suggest then that IFN (interferon) may stimulate the production of small amounts of H2O2 and possibly other oxygen intermediates (OH) which are a necessary event early in the pathway of IFN activation of human NK cells."

Note: Data retrieved from the Medical College of Wisconsin indicates that some forms of cancer are resistant to H2O2 therapy (insufficient catalase?). Data is not presently available to be certain which types of cancer are susceptible and which types are resistant. In one local case, it was not effective on Leukemia.

## The Gerson Primer and Cancer

Cancer patients who want to benefit from the past 50 years of research and experiences of the Gerson Institute are well advised to obtain a copy of **"The Gerson Primer."** You can obtain it by calling 619-585-7600 or writing to The Gerson Institute, PO Box 430, Bonita, CA 91908.

## Friendly Flora and Natural Killer Cell Function

From my own observations, cancer and other conditions like candidiasis exist when there is a failure of intestinal health and an *absence of friendly intestinal flora* along with a loss of *Natural Killer Cell activity*. It has already been demonstrated that a high fiber diet and increased butyrate production from bifido bacteria in the colon can help prevent colon cancer. Restoring intestinal health and a normal functioning immune system are related events and prevent the reoccurrence of cancers.

Natural Killer cells are a type of white blood cells that search out and destroy cancer cells. A **Natural Killer Cytotoxic Activity Test** is available through your physician. Specialty Labs and ImmunoSciences Labs (310-657-1077 or 800-950-4686) both provide this test. Natural Killer cell function is not a "count" of the number of NK cells your have but rather a measure of the ability of this type of white blood cell to destroy (lyse) cancer cells in a lab.

The die off (lyse) of cancer cell is measured in "**lytic**" units. Normal people have from 35 to 250 "lytic" units. When cancer exists, lytic units are usually 20 or less and often in the single digits. When "lytic" units are 50 or higher, cancer rarely exists. Another useful test is "**albumin levels**". Cancer may exist when they are below normal but rarely when they are at normal levels. *Vegetarian digestive enzymes taken with meals can help raise albumin levels.* For information on how to restore Natural Killer cell activity, read the book called **"Immune Restoration Handbook"** by Mark Konlee. Information about this book can be found at **www.keephopealive.org**.

Infusion therapy of either H2O2 or Ozone Autohemotherapy of the blood must be done by a physician trained in Bio-oxidative therapies.

# Chapter IV

## Hydrogen Peroxide - Safety Considerations

35% Hydrogen Peroxide solution must never be poured into a clear unlabeled container or stored in a refrigerator. Some people have had tragic accidents by mistaking the 35% $H_2O_2$ solution for plain water. Ingesting straight 35% $H_2O_2$ can cause irreparable damage to a weak stomach. An overdose can even cause death from blood alkalosis and by depleting sugar reserves or by foaming in the blood causing a gas bubble that stops blood from circulating. This only happens if too much $H_2O_2$ enters the blood too quickly. **Read warning on the back cover of this book before purchasing or using 35% $H_2O_2$ solution.** Anyone with a weak stomach should not use hydrogen peroxide orally in any form.

## $H_2O_2$ and Oxidative Stress

$H_2O_2$ usually brings significant results when 50 drops a day or 35% $H_2O_2$ (the equivalent being about 7 teaspoons of a 6% solution) or more are assimilated into the body. The highest dosage I ever heard of anyone taking was 100 drops a day orally. I would not recommend this high a dose on a continuous basis due to the oxidative stress on healthy cells. If the immune system has high levels of white blood cells and high levels of Neutrophils, the use of $H_2O_2$ probably would not provide much additional benefit as Neutrophils produce $H_2O_2$. $H_2O_2$, like ozone, can be of life saving benefit when the immune system is not functioning at par.

## $H_2O_2$ and iron – a bad combination

For several years, I was puzzled why some people could take $H_2O_2$ orally with water and report benefits and no adverse effects while others reported a sore stomach syndrome. Recently, I received a letter from a person who told how he thought he nearly ruined his stomach drinking hydrogen peroxide with well water that was high in iron. He reported no adverse effects from taking $H_2O_2$ orally after he switched to distilled water. An abstract from the Medical College of Wisconsin reports that iron in the presence of $H_2O_2$ will produce Superoxide radicals. Iron by itself will produce Superoxide radicals that can damage the stomach mucosa. In the presence of iron or copper, the production of these

Superoxide radicals increases. Therefore, to avoid this problem, use distilled water or Reverse Osmosis water only when taking H2O2 orally. Do not use well water or tap water which may contain iron and avoid any foods or vitamin supplements with iron for both 1 hour before or after taking H2O2 orally.
Note: The CDC reported that iron supplements caused the death of 11 children in 1992 due to damage to the stomach membranes. It is safest to obtain your iron from natural sources. Your safest source of iron is blackstrap molasses which is also high in calcium and potassium and some 50 trace minerals. It may be used 1 to 2 hours before or after taking H2O2 orally. Other food sources high in iron are oatmeal, sunflower seeds, seafood (fish) and dark green vegetables.

## An important request to Health Food Store owners and health care professionals

35% H2O2 should be handled by and sold only to health care professionals. Please keep 35% H2O2 off store shelves and in the back room for health care professionals. However, if you feel you must sell 35% H2O2 solution to your customers, I would advise for safety reasons to limit the amount to 2 to 4 ounces and place it in a brown glass bottle with a dropper pipette. Advise them to store this in a freezer until it is used. A small bottle stored in a freezer is good for at least 10 years.

**For most purposes (food grade quality) H2O2 solution of 6% or 7% should only be made available to the public.** *Everyone who buys hydrogen peroxide (food grade quality) should have a copy of this book to know how to properly and safely use the product.* Ask your H2O2 supplier to provide you with a 6% or 7% H2O2 solution. If you cannot locate a source of 6% H2O2 solution, write to us and we will help find a source for you.

The US government lists H2O2 solutions of 8% concentration or less as non-hazardous and those above 8% as hazardous.

## Anti-oxidants and Bio-oxidative therapies

For anyone using H2O2 in any form or ozone for more than 30 days or any person who is in a generally weakened state, the use of anti-oxidants is recommended to protect healthy cells from oxidative stress. Anti-oxidants strengthen the cell membranes and protect against damage caused by free radicals. Free radicals are molecules with unpaired electrons in their outer ring and damage cell membranes by stealing electrons from the membranes of healthy cells. Synthetic Vitamin C (chemically made from corn) sold almost everywhere, should be avoided as studies find it will damage the DNA in the cells. No such evidence exists for natural vitamin C.

The following is a list of the most important anti-oxidants and suggested adult dosages. Natural Vitamin C only – Acerola cherries (4 grams daily) or Camu Camu – 2 grams daily dried fruit powder yields about 500 mg Vitamin C. Pycnogenol - 30 mg - 3 to 5 times daily; or use Elderberry or Bilberry extract, Vitamin A – Cod Liver Oil – 1 or 2 teaspoons daily; Beta-carotene - 50 to 100 mg daily; Pure cranberry juice – 4 to 6 ozs daily – highest in free radical quenching activity of all fruits.

For selenium, use Brazil nuts and fish or use high selenium mustard greens. Take at least 400 mcg daily of these food based sources of selenium. Do not use L-selenomethionine as this is made in a laboratory, is not food based, and can have serious side effects including transitory stroke. Avoid one-a-day vitamin tablets as these are polluted with synthetic vitamins. High doses of synthetic vitamins in pills or in breakfast cereal (i.e Total breakfast cereal) are foreign and toxic to the body. Buy whole foods only (Chlorella, Spirulina, wheat germ, Royal jelly, desiccated liver, Brewers yeast etc) that are high in natural vitamin and mineral complexes. Cold-processed whey proteins like Immunocal or ImmunoPro and CoQ10 from sardines, broccoli, spinach, kale and other dark green vegetables.

Anti-oxidants should be taken 24 hours or more before or after the use of H2O2 and other oxidative therapies like ozone. Otherwise, the anti-oxidants may cancel out the benefits of the oxidative therapies. **Antioxidants (in pill form including vitamin C) should not be used with chemotherapy or the chemotherapy simply won't work.** Many forms of chemotherapy work by causing oxidative reactions that destroy the tumors and some synthetic anti-oxidants interfere with these reactions. Wholesome foods with naturally occurring antioxidants are not a problem because of the natural synergy that exists in whole foods with multiple ingredients. Wholesome foods (whole grains and vegetables) are very beneficial regardless of what kind of therapy you choose.

Natural sources of Vitamin C like Rose hips, Acerola cherries, Camu Camu, Amla and oranges may be used daily and are an effective source of Vitamin C. *Obtaining most of your vitamin supplements in lower doses from whole food sources is more beneficial than taking synthetic mega-vitamin pills,* a habit that will eventually cause mineral deficiencies. Some synthetic vitamins and amino acid chelates have defective molecular structures and cannot be used by the cells and become toxic waste products.

# Catalase

Catalase is the enzyme in the body that breaks down hydrogen peroxide into water and oxygen. One vegetable high in catalase is raw potatoes. A science experiment at the University of Wisconsin in Madison shows the release of oxygen from the surface of a slice of potato placed in a glass of $H_2O_2$. A raw potato eaten after oral ingestion of $H_2O_2$ probably would have the same effect in the stomach breaking down the hydrogen peroxide into water and releasing oxygen gas.

# Alkalosis

I have also found that a small quantity of $H_2O_2$ with water moves urine and saliva pH in an alkaline direction. One of the side effects of oral hydrogen peroxide is that it lowers production of hydrochloric acid which is why it should not be used at meal times. The best time to take $H_2O_2$ is on an empty stomach (1/2 hr or more hour before meals) or 2 or 3 hours after your last meal.

Alkalosis is a condition that can be determined when you add the pH values of both urine and saliva pH and divide by 2. If the number is higher than 6.4, you are too alkaline. Alkalosis can create problems as bad as acidosis. Alkalosis can be caused by too much $H_2O_2$, germanium, CO Q10, aspirins and a vegetarian or fruit diet that is too low in amino acids. In the event of alkalosis, the use of these supplements should be reduced and the diet should be adjusted to contain more amino acids (yogurt, proteins, legumes, fish) and complex carbohydrates from gluten-free grains like brown and wild rice, corn, amaranth and quinoa.

Vitamin C or apple cider vinegar will help counter the effects of alkalosis and will temporarily lower saliva pH when it is too high. Alkalosis is associated with allergies and slow digestion

# Chapter V
# Bio-Oxidative Formulas

In this book, I am releasing several formulas for making your own Bio-oxidative medicines. Some formulas are designed for persons to make at home and others for health care professionals. The 3% Peroxy Spray work equally as well as the Peroxy Gel. Peroxy Spray should be stored in a refrigerator if not used on a regular basis. Either may be left out at room temperature for several days at a time. However, they will gradually lose their potency if exposed continuously to warm temperatures for more than two weeks at a time.

## Health benefits from using Peroxy Gel or Spray

a. Aching Joints
b. Arthritis
c. Rheumatism
d. Pain (lessens or eliminates altogether)
e. Back Massage
f. Athlete's foot
g. Sore muscles
h. Burns
i. Bruises
j. Minor infections
k. Rashes
l. Insect bites
m. Fungal and yeast infections.
n. Carpal tunnel syndrome

Several letters received by us from customers indicate that Peroxy Gel is also beneficial for -

1. Skin cancer
2. Tumors
3. Gangrene
4. Improves circulation in hands and feet - restores feeling.
5. Cuts and wounds that won't heal
6. Pleurisy (followed by a heat pad)
7. Emphysema

Testimonial letters tell of some incredible stories of healing experiences and of the gratitude people experience from using the gel.

Several letters claim hydrogen peroxide was effective against skin cancer and tumors near the surface of the skin As a topical application, it is believed to be compatible with any other treatment prescribed by your physician. Dosages: Massage up to two tablespoons daily into the skin or use the 3% Peroxy Spray.

## For Home Use
### 3% Peroxy Spray (for external use)
(Formula for one pint)

1. Into a bowl, pour 1 cup of aloe vera juice and add one cup of a 6% or 7% Hydrogen Peroxide solution. Mix with a spatula and pour into a bottle with a spray nozzle like an old Windex bottle. Keep refrigerated when not in use. For external use, spray directly on to any area of the body you desire. Keep out of eyes. Use the same as you would Peroxy Gel.
2. Label the bottle "Peroxy Spray - 3% H2O2 solution".
3. For a 1.5% H2O2 solution, mix one cup of 3% H2O2 solution (from the brown bottle – drugstore variety) with one cup of aloe vera juice and mark it H2O2 and Aloe solution for external use.

Note: *Do not* place 3% Peroxy Spray in the eyes. Some people have mixed the 3% solution with equal amounts of aloe vera juice and used a few drops for infections in the ears.

**DO NOT USE H2O2 OR PEROXY SPRAY ON HERPES INFECTIONS, COLD SORES OR SHINGLES.** H2O2 may actually stimulate the herpes virus. Instead, try lemon oil. Patchouli oil or Lomatium dissectum tincture topically. Also apply ice cubes topically or for use freshly made ozonated olive oil. (See instructions in last chapter on ozone).

## For home use - Sublingual H2O2

1. Mix 2 tablespoons of 6% or 8% H2O2 (food grade quality) with 4 tablespoons of Aloe Vera juice. This gives you about 2% H2O2 solution in aloe vera juice. Using a Dropper Pipette, take 20 (1/4 teaspoon.) to 40 drops (1/2 teaspoon) under the tongue every 30 to 60 minutes or as directed by a health care professional who can monitor the effects and advise you. Hold solution in the mouth for 3 minutes until most of it is absorbed and then drink a full glass of water. Use up to 1/2 hour before meals but no earlier than 2 hours after a meal. You can also rinse your mouth with this solution and gargle with it also.

**NOTICE**: Do not use hydrogen peroxide orally on a continuous basis as it acts like an intestinal antibiotic and will kill off friendly flora. Think of it more as a low cost antibiotic (drug) and not a dietary supplement. H2O2 is a poor mans medicine. Use sublingually for 2 weeks for non life-threatening conditions. If the problem persist, see a physician. Small amounts applied topically may be used daily on a continuous basis if needed. If the need is continuous, seek professional help.

The **aloe vera acts like a carrier** helping the H2O2 penetrate faster into the tissues and into the blood vessels. It also **buffers** the solution making it gentler on the mucus membranes and more patient friendly.

## The remaining formulas listed here are for Health Care Professionals Only

### 6% Peroxy Spray – a very good choice

(Formula for one pint of a 6% hydrogen peroxide solution)
1. Into a bowl, pour 1 and 1/3 cup of aloe vera juice. To this add 1/3 cup of glycerin and 1/3 cup of 35% H2O2. Mix with a spatula and pour into a bottle with a spray nozzle like an old Windex bottle. Keep refrigerated when not in use. For external use, spray directly on to any area of the body you desire. Keep out of eyes. Use the same as you would Peroxy Gel. Label the bottle "Peroxy Spray - 6% H2O2 solution". The Spray is easier to make than the gel and works just as well. In fact it absorbs more easily.

### 6% Peroxy Gel
### Formula for one pint
<u>For external use only</u>

1. Into a bowl squeeze 1 and 1/3 cups of aloe vera gelly. (Obtain from a health food store or drug store). Make sure you buy an aloe vera grade gel that is thick and solid for best results.

2. In a separate bowl mix 1/3 cup of glycerin with 1/3 cup of 35% hydrogen peroxide solution. Use a spatula to mix the two together. (35% H2O2 can be obtained from a health food store or look in the Yellow Page Phone directory under "Chemicals" or see addresses at the end of these instructions. Glycerin can be obtained from a drug store or look in the Yellow Page Phone directory under "Chemicals" or see addresses at the end of this book).

3. Pour the glycerin and 35% H2O2 solution mixture into the bowl containing the Aloe Vera Gel. Use a spatula and gently stir all these ingredients together. At first it will look soupy for about a minute, then as you keep stirring, it will thicken and turn into a nice thick absorbable

gel. Use a spoon or the spatula to pour the Peroxy Gel into an empty wide mouth mayonnaise jar.

4. Do not try to pour the gel into a small neck bottle, as you will likely have difficulty getting the thick mixture to pour. Store your Peroxy Gel in a refrigerator when you are not using it. Mark a blank label "Peroxy Gel" "For External use Only - 6% H2O2. " Enjoy your new product. Each teaspoon of Peroxy Gel contains the equivalent of 15 drops of 35% H2O2. This 6% Peroxy Gel is the same concentration as the original formula we sold to thousands of satisfied customers.

## 3% Peroxy Gel
(Formula for one pint)

3% Peroxy Gel is used where a mild formula is needed for sensitive areas like burns or cuts. To make a 3% gel, add 1 and 1/2 cups of aloe vera gelly to a bowl. Add 1/3 cup of glycerin and 3 Tablespoons of 35% H2O2. Stir together with a spatula and pour into a wide mouth jar. Keep refrigerated when not in use.

## H2O2 and Aloe Vera solution for Sublingual use

Mix **one part 35% (food grade) H2O2** solution with **17 parts aloe vera juice** to make a finished product that has 2% H2O2 in solution. Always try to find aloe vera juice with the fewest preservatives or preferably, none at all. For adults, 20 to 40 drops under the tongue every 30 to 60 minutes and no later than 30 minutes before eating or earlier than 2 hours after meals. Example: 8 am Breakfast. 10 am - sublingual H2O2, 10:30 or 11 am sublingual solution; 11:30 or 12 noon - sublingual H2O2 solution. 12:30 p.m. - lunch. Patient may resume sublingual applications of H2O2 solution after 2:30 pm. For children, reduce dosage according to body weight.

**Skin Cancer:** With a Q-tip, apply straight 35% H2O2 solution to the skin cancer two or 3 times daily. For clients who need to apply 35% H2O2 solution at home, give then 35% H2O2 solution is a 2 ounce bottle with a child proof cap and a dropper pipette and/or Q tips. Instruct them to keep it in a freezer only - out of reach of children. By dispensing it only in very small quantities, accidents can be avoided or minimized.

# Chapter VI
# History of Medical Ozone
by John Pittman M.D.

Ozone (O3) is an energized form of oxygen with extra electrons present, which spontaneously disperse from the molecule as soon as they are produced. About eighty years ago, it was discovered that ozone could be used to disinfect wounds and surfaces. This was later found be due to the effect of these electrons blasting holes through the membranes of viruses, bacteria, yeast, and abnormal tissue cells.

German researchers have been leaders in the development of ozone technology. One of the first uses of ozone was in the 1930's, when it was found to be effective in treating various types of inflammatory bowel disorders, such as ulcerative colitis, Crohn's disease and chronic bacterial diarrhea. In this procedure, ozone gas is delivered into the rectum through a catheter tip, where it is absorbed through the lining of the colon.

The Germans later developed a technique for treating blood with ozone called "major autohemotherapy." In this procedure, about 300 cc's of blood is taken from a vein into a vacuum bottle. Ozone is then bubbled through the blood, after which the blood is reinfused. In this procedure, ozone destroys any virus particles in the blood. It is also absorbed into the plasma and after re-infusion, disperses throughout the body. Another technique for using ozone is direct infusion, in which ozone gas is injected directly into the vein. This has the advantage of being more precise in terms of dosage. delivered, as well as allowing administration of higher concentrations. Other techniques include direct application to the skin through the use of ozone baths, as well as minor autohemotherapy, in which blood and ozone are mixed in a small syringe and injected intramuscularly into the buttock. Through further work, the Germans were able to determine that ozone was incredibly effective in destroying such infections as hepatitis, Epstein-Barr virus, herpes, cytomegalovirus and HIV. With the realization that HIV was susceptible to ozone, the Germans began using the autohemotherapy technique to treat AIDS patients as soon as this was a recognized disease.

There have been numerous anecdotes about the German's success with ozone, and many physicians in this country have also been using it with great success. Until recently, neither government institutions nor private corporations have sponsored any rigid clinical ozone studies. There appears to be a built-in bias against the development of therapies such as ozone, because it is a non-patentable gas. Our pharmaceutical industry has developed based on the ability to patent synthetic drugs that can be sold at a profit, and thus recoup the initial investment expense. This has resulted in a system that supports drug development by this method and has discouraged the development of simple, inexpensive or non-patentable substances. Nevertheless, numerous physicians have used ozone successfully, and have risked sanctions by federal and state authorities, as this is not an FDA approved treatment.

Note: Dr. John Pittman, M.D. can be reached at 4505 Fair Meadow Ln, No 111, Raleigh, N.C. 27607. Ph No. 919-571-4391

## Ozone in Nature

by Saul Pressman

In nature, there is a cycle of oxygen just like there is a cycle of water. Oxygen is released from plants on land and plankton in the sea during photosynthesis. The oxygen is lighter than air and floats upward in the atmosphere. At the 20-30 km region, strong ultraviolet radiation in the 185-200 nanometer wavelength bombards the oxygen and turns some of it into ozone. The ozone created exists as a thin layer in the atmosphere and it blocks out the small portion of the UV spectrum that it absorbs. The great majority of the UV reaches the earth allowing sun-tanning, which Dr. Michael Carpendale of the San Francisco Veteran's Administration Hospital has noted is useful in a very efficacious therapy developed in the early years of this century. We hear a great deal about the thinning of the ozone layer in the media, but the facts are otherwise.

Ozone production in the upper atmosphere is dependent on the amount of energy coming from the sun. During peaks of solar activity, ozone is created at a greater rate. During lulls in the sunspot cycle, the ozone layer is thinner. The lowest level ever measured was in 1962. At night, on the dark side of the planet, the ozone layer disappears, in a few hours. The layer is reformed as the sun rises in the morning. There is no ozone over the poles in the winter because there is no sunlight. Chlorofluorocarbons are the heaviest and most inert compound gases possible and are totally harmless -- ask any refrigerant expert.

Ozone is produced constantly in the upper atmosphere as long as the sun is shining, and since ozone is heavier than air, it begins to fall earthward. As it falls, it combines with any pollutant it contacts, cleaning the air -- nature's wonderful self-cleaning system. If ozone contacts water vapor as it falls, it forms hydrogen peroxide, a component of rainwater, and the reason why rainwater causes plants to grow better than irrigation. Ozone is also created by lightning, and the amount produced in an average storm is often triple the allowable limit of .015 PPM as set by the US EPA. This ozone is what gives the air the wonderful fresh smell after a rain, and is of the highest benefit to anyone fortunate enough to be breathing it.

Ozone is also created by waterfalls and crashing surf, which accounts for the energetic feeling and calm experienced near these sites. Another way ozone is produced is by photons from the sun breaking apart nitrous oxide, a pollutant formed by the combustion of hydrocarbons in the internal combustion engine. This ozone can accumulate in smog due to temperature inversions and is a lung and eye irritant. These are the forms of ozone created by natural processes in the atmosphere.

## Ozone since 1857

The first ozone generators were developed by Werner von Siemens in Germany in 1857, and 1870 saw the first report on ozone being used therapeutically to purify blood, by C. Lender in Germany.

There is evidence of the use of ozone as a disinfectant from 1881, mentioned by Dr. Kellogg in his book on diphtheria. In October of 1893, the world's first water treatment plant using ozone was installed in Ousbaden, Holland, and today there are over 3000 municipalities around the world that use ozone to clean their water and sewage. In 1885, the Florida Medical Association published "Ozone" by Dr. Charles J. Kenworth, MD, detailing the use of ozone for therapeutic purposes.

In September 1896, the electrical genius Nikola Tesla patented his first ozone generator, and in 1900, he formed the Tesla Ozone Company. Tesla sold ozone machines to doctors for medical use, the same thing we are doing 100 years later, with a design based on one of his from the 1920s. We have seen one of these 75-year-old generators, and it still works perfectly. Tesla produced ozonated olive oil and sold it to naturopaths, and we do, too.

In 1898, the Institute for Oxygen Therapy was started in Berlin by Thauerkauf and Luth. They injected ozone into animals and bonded ozone to magnesium, producing Homozon. Beginning in 1898, Dr. Benedict Lust, a German doctor practicing in New York, who was the originator and founder Naturopathy, wrote many articles and books on ozone. In 1902, J.H. Clarke's "A Dictionary of Practical Materia Medica," London describes the successful use of ozonated water in treating anemia, cancer, diabetes, influenza, morphine poisoning, canker sores, strychnine poisoning and whooping cough. In 1911,

"A Working Manual of High Frequency Currents" was published by Dr. Noble Eberhart, MD. Dr. Eberhart was head of the Department of Physiologic Therapeutics at Loyola University. He used ozone to treat tuberculosis, anemia, chlorosis, tinnitus, whooping cough, asthma, bronchitis, hay fever, insomnia, pneumonia, diabetes, gout and syphilis.

In 1913, the Eastern Association for Oxygen Therapy was formed by Dr. Blass and some German associates. During World War 1, ozone was used to treat wounds, trench foot, gangrene and the effects of poison gas. Dr. Albert Wolff of Berlin also used ozone for colon cancer, cervical cancer and ulcers in 1915.

In 1920, Dr. Charles Neiswanger, MD, the President of the Chicago Hospital College of Medicine published "Electro Therapeutical Practice." Chapter 32 was entitled " Ozone as a Therapeutic Agent."

In 1926, Dr. Otto Warburg of the Kaiser Institute in Berlin announced that the cause of cancer is lack of oxygen at the cellular level. He received the Nobel Prize for Medicine in 1931 and again in 1944, the only person to ever receive two Nobel Prizes for Medicine. He was also nominated for a third.

In 1929, a book called "Ozone and Its Therapeutic Action" was published in the US listing 114 diseases and how to treat them with ozone. Its authors were the heads of all the leading American hospitals.

In 1933, the American Medical Association, headed up by Dr. Simmons set out to destroy all medical treatments that were competitive to drug therapy. The suppression of ozone therapy began then, and it continues in the US to this day.

The Swiss dentist E.A. Fisch was using ozone in dentistry before 1932, and introduced it to the German surgeon Erwin Payr who used it from that time forward. Aubourg and Lacoste were French physicians using ozone insufflation from 1934-1938.

In 1948, Dr. William Turska of Oregon began using ozone, employing a machine of his own design, and in 1951, Dr. Turska wrote the article "Oxidation" which is still relevant today, and is included in our booklet. Dr. Turska pioneered injection of ozone into the portal vein, thereby reaching the liver.

From 1953 onward, German doctor Hans Wolff used ozone in his practice, writing the book "Medical Ozone," and training many doctors in ozone therapy. In 1957, Dr. J. Hansler patented an ozone generator that has formed the basis of the German expansion of ozone therapy over the last 35 years. Today over 7000 German doctors use ozone therapy daily.

In 1961, Hans Wolff introduced the techniques of major and minor autohemotherapy. In 1977, Dr. Renate Viebahn provided a technical overview of ozone action in the body. In 1979, Dr. George Freibott began treating his first AIDS patient with ozone, and in 1980, Dr. Horst Kief also reported success in treating AIDS with ozone. In 1987, Dr. Rilling and Dr. Viebahn published "The Use of Ozone in Medicine," the standard text on the subject. In 1990, the Cubans reported on their success in treating glaucoma, conjunctivitis and retinitis pigmentosa with ozone. In 1992, the Russians revealed their techniques of using ozone bubbled into brine to treat burn victims with astounding results.

Today, after 125 years of usage, ozone therapy is a recognized modality in many nations: Germany, France, Italy, Russia, Romania, Czech Republic, Poland, Hungary, Bulgaria, Israel, Cuba, Japan, Mexico, and in five US states.

## Types of Ozone Generators

Oxygen is the only gas that will pick up and hold electrical energy. In doing so, it becomes tremendously active and seeks to combine with all other substances. The list of substances that are inert to ozone is very short, and includes glass, Teflon, Kynar, silicone and gold. Therefore, any ozone generator and auxiliary equipment must be composed of these substances only. There are several different techniques used to produce medical grade ozone, where freedom from contamination is critical.

One type of generator uses an ultraviolet lamp as its source. It produces a very small amount of ozone in a narrow frequency bandwidth of ultraviolet light. Outside of that bandwidth, UV destroys ozone. A UV lamp is unreliable because it is subject to degradation over time, causing uncertainty regarding concentration, and eventually it burns out.

The second method of ozone production is corona discharge, where a tube with a hot cathode is surrounded by a screen anode. The best ones are called dual-dielectric, because they have a layer of glass separating each component from the gas stream. This prevents contamination of the ozone in the best designs, but heat is produced, and heat destroys ozone. To compensate for the loss in concentration, more electricity is used, resulting in more heat, and consequent electrical failure. This produces generators that have short lives.

Lack of durability has always beset the ozone generator industry, and was one of the major reasons for naturopaths mostly abandoning ozone therapy during the Thirties. I have spoken to doctors who have used ozone for three decades and have gone through a half dozen generators in that time, due to the lack of a durable generator, and reliable servicing. Fortunately, there is a third method of producing clean, medical grade ozone. That method is called cold plasma. It uses two glass rods filled with a noble gas, electrostatic plasma field that turns the oxygen into ozone. Since there is no appreciable current, no heat is produced. Thus the generator will last a very long time, limited only by the quality of the power supply. The original cold plasma ozone generators were invented by Nikola Tesla in the 1920s, and they still work 75 years later.

### Ozone Therapy is Safest Known Therapy

Ozone has been found to be an extremely safe medical therapy, free from side effects. In a 1980 study done by the German Medical Society for Ozone Therapy, 644 therapists were polled regarding their 384,775 patients, comprising a total of 5,579,238 ozone treatments administered. There were only 40 cases of side effects noted out of this number that represents the incredibly low rate of .000007%, and only four fatalities. Ozone has thus proven to be the safest medical therapy ever devised.

### Dosage and Frequency

When it comes to dosage and frequency of administration, there is some difference of opinion. Dr. Carpendale believes that a high concentration is necessary to kick-start the immune system initially, followed by much lower concentrations. He believes that continued high concentrations may be immunosuppressive, based on T-4 cell counts. Other doctors, such as Dr. Turska, recommend initial medium concentration doses, three times per week, followed by twice weekly at lower concentration, followed by weekly injection as long as necessary. Dr. Stan Beyrle recommends injection every four days at medium concentration.
    Dr. Wang has been giving daily injections at medium concentration, and direct injection into breast tumors. Dr. Freibott recommends very high concentrations at low dosages, with the emphasis on observing the patient's blood saturation.
    Dr. Rillings classic, ***The Use of Ozone in Medicine***, recently reprinted, gives many recommendations on dosage and concentration. There is no evidence that long-**term** treatment on a daily basis has any detrimental effect. Doctors who have used it for decades have only positive results to report. Ozone is blatantly non-toxic. There is no

evidence of free radical damage; in fact, ozone is the best free radical scavenger there is.

Ozone also stimulates production of superoxide dismutase, catalase, and glutathione peroxidase, which are the enzymes in the cell wall that protect the cell from free radical damage, so ozone actually helps prevent free radical damage. Dr. Horst Kief of Germany recommends taking Vitamin A and Vitamin E supplements when receiving ozone treatments.

It is know that Vitamin C is antagonistic to ozone, and persons taking mega doses of Vitamin C should maintain a 12-hour spread between ingestion and the ozone treatment, although ozone does not break down Vitamin C in the body. This effect of Vitamin C can be used to advantage in intravenous administration. Sometimes a patient will have a lot of coughing caused by ozone out gassing in the lungs from having had a bit too much too fast from the IV. If the coughing continues longer than 30 minutes, it can be stopped by administering 5000 mg of Vitamin C orally.

The ozone reaction will end quickly and the patient will be more comfortable and have a better attitude toward the therapy. The rate of injection should be very slow, about 10 cc per minute. Since intravenous injections are 95-98 % oxygen and 2-5 % ozone gas, some doctors have expressed concern about embolism. However, there is no danger of embolism from injections of oxygen and ozone. Only nitrogen forms a dangerous gas bubble, as when divers get the bends from surfacing too fast. The human body runs perfectly well on 100% oxygen; consider the fighter pilots who breathe 100% oxygen daily for years -- they have the highest reflexes, visual acuity and level of general health of any group of humans.

## Magnets unclump red blood cells

Doctors have reported that they can enhance ozone therapy by using magnet therapy simultaneously. Permanent magnets can be used with the north pole facing upward, toward the patient, on the underside of the treatment table. Magnets cause a polarization of red blood cells, which have iron in them. The polarization causes red blood cells to unclump and become more flexible, so that they can bend and get through the finest capillaries, improving microcirculation and preventing literally hundreds of diseases. Therefore, there is a synergistic effect between ozone and magnets.

## Ozone and water in the body

The human body is 2/3 water. Of that, 90% is lymph and 10% is blood. The cell functions by burning sugar in oxygen to provide energy. The waste products are carbon dioxide and water. If there is insufficient oxygen at the cellular level, the burn will be incomplete, and carbon monoxide and lactic acid will be formed. The body cannot easily rid itself of monoxide; it prevents hemoglobin from picking up fresh oxygen, and the body temperature is lowered. The lactic acid will build up in the system, clogging the nerve pathways, eventually calcifying and causing degeneration. More oxygen is required to come in and oxidize these toxins, but if it is not available, they build up. The blood will carry a heavy load of sludge, and toxins will be deposited in the fat. The water that composes the body gets dirtier and dirtier. Disease is the result.

This is where ozone shines -- in eliminating toxicity from the body. Ozone taken on a daily basis will, over time, clean all the fluid of the body, safely. Ozone has been used to clean water for large cities for over 100 years. The water **engineers** have a value that they use to measure the effectiveness of ozone in cleaning water. This is the CT value. It is a product of concentration x time. (CxT)

## Ozonated Water

For prevention, a major benefit can be derived from regularly drinking ozonated water. Water is a fascinating substance, and we all take it for granted. Chemically it is considered to be an oxygen atom bound with two hydrogen atoms. The bond angle between the two hydrogen atoms is known to be variable, depending on the amount of energy in the molecule. Research has shown that water whose bond angle is 101 degrees is 'dead' water, bereft of life-giving energy. When water is distilled the bond angle expands to 120 degrees upon evaporation, but collapses to 101 degrees upon condensation, and is therefore dead. A bond angle of 103 degrees corresponds to average water.

A bond angle of 106 degrees produces activated, energized water, and is attainable by placing a magnet, north pole inward, against the water container. The highest energy obtainable in liquid water is a bond angle of 109.5 degrees, and this is attainable only ozonating water at 4 degrees C. Ozone will not stay in water for very long, even at 4 degrees C. To hold the ozone in the water over long periods, it is necessary to add a few drops of Concentrate, which is a solution of trace minerals from the Great Salt Lake with the sodium, cadmium, copper and lead removed.

The ozone hangs on to the minerals without oxidizing them and remains available over many months. In general, un-mineralized water should not be consumed. Drink water that has gone through reverse osmosis, carbon filtering, and is then ozonated. There are some contaminants that will pass through R/O and carbon, such as fluorine. Ozonating the water removes all such contaminants and energizes the water until the bond angle reaches 109.5 degrees. Ozonate water for 15 minutes per liter, about five minutes per glass.

## Ozonating the Lymph

Women have an advantage, in that vaginal insufflation requires no preparation, and can be administered for very long periods of time, hours in fact. The gas will usually find its way into the uterus, out the Fallopian tubes, and then into the abdominal cavity.

Liver problems and pelvic inflammatory disease (PID) can be addressed in this way. This is also a good way of getting ozone into the lymph system. For men, cleaning the lymph system is not as easy, and requires use of a body suit or a steam cabinet. The body suit is a less that popular aesthetic experience.

The Saunette steam cabinet, however, is a pleasurable experience. Because of the moist heat, the pores are open, and the capillaries are dilated. The ozone enters and oxidizes toxins in the fat, the lymph and the blood. The skin is the largest organ of elimination. The person sweats the oxidized toxins back out, avoiding the dump of toxins to the liver and colon that can bring on the symptoms of toxic shock overload. Instead, the person emerges from the steam cabinet feeling extremely relaxed and mellow, and ready for bed. This is an ideal way of counteracting the stress of the day.

## What does Ozone do?

Ozone: inactivates viruses, bacteria, yeast, fungus and protozoa. stimulates the immune system cleans arteries and veins, improves circulation, purifies the blood and lymph, normalizes hormone and enzyme production, reduces inflammation, reduces pain, calms the nerves, stops bleeding, prevents shock, prevents stroke damage, reduces cardiac arrhythmia, improves brain function and memory, oxidizes toxins, allowing their excretion, chelates heavy metals; it works well in conjunction with EDTA prevents and reverses degenerative diseases prevents and treats communicable diseases prevents and eliminates autoimmune diseases.

The following articles on ozone are found on this website – www.ozonio.com.br

The Cause and Prevention of Cancer Saul Pressman
Superoxygenation for Health Saul Pressman
Ozone and Free Radicals Waves Forrest
Free Radicals, Ozone and antioxidants Dr. Horst Kief
Free Radical Pathology Chelation Therapy
Free Radical Theory Dr. Deepak Chopra
Oxidation Dr. George Freibott
Oxidation Dr. William Turska
Ozone Therapy Fritz Schellander
Ozone: Its Therapeutic Action
Better Blood Sterilization With Ozone Canadian Govt
Are Worry-Free Transfusions Just a Whiff of Ozone Away? Albert Baggs
The Importance of Oxygen Dr. Robert E. Willner
The Healing Crisis 'Alive' Magazine
Interesting Medical Ozone Facts Dr. H.E. Sartori
AIDS and Cancer are Curable Dr. George Freibott
The History of Medical Ozone in the Treatment of AIDS Dr. John Pittman
Immunization and Ozone Saul Pressman
Contemporary Ozone Applications Dr. Kurt Donsbach
MSM: Methyl Sulfonyl Methane Saul Pressman
Methylene Blue Saul Pressman
Flax Oil and Ozone
Hydrogen Peroxide Walter Grotz
So You're Thinking About Trying Ozone David Sterling
Protocols of Ozone Administration Dr. Ziegfried Rilling
Direct IV Injection of Ozone Dr. J. Pittman
Major Autohemotherapy Protocol Dr. F. Shallenberger
Using Ozone in the Home
Ozone Has Been Used to Treat Dr. H.E.
Suggested Protocols Dr. William Turska
Ozone and Its Uses in Medical Therapy Dr. Robert E. Willner
Ozone Applications Brad Hunter, P.Eng
Healing Ozone - Phoebe Chow, ND (Alive magazine #156 Oct./95)
Ozone Books

For copies of the rest of the articles listed here, visit this website – **www.ozonio.com.br** to download the rest of this free Internet book. If the event this website should ever become unavailable, I have saved in Microsoft "Word" format a copy of the book on a floppy disc in PC or MAC format and copies are available.

Note: Author's comment. I do not agree with all the views published on this website about the therapeutic benefits of ozone as some writers have made exaggerated claims but I do substantially agree with the majority of what is written here.

**Physicians**: The International Bio-Oxidative Medicine Foundation has merged with ACAM - the American College for the Advancement of Medicine (**www.acamnet.org**). This progressive organization provides information for health care professionals and training in the use of bio-oxidative therapies, edta chelation therapies, herbal and holistic medicine and other progressive treatments. ACAM's phone number is 800-532-3688.

Physicians wanting a reference book on technical information on how to administer ozone should obtain a copy of *THE USE OF OZONE IN MEDICINE* (ISBN 3-7760-1481-4), by R. Viebahn Ph.D. (translated from German). Check with Amazon.com and other Internet book sources for a new or used copy. Search words: "Ozone" or "hydrogen peroxide" for other fine books like one by William C. Douglass M.D., Nathaniel Altman and others.

Information on how to use ozone in a more limited capacity for home use is found in a book on immune-based nutritional therapies called **"Immune Restoration Handbook"**, ($24.95 postpaid Write: Keep Hope Alive, P.O. Box 270041, West Allis, WI 53227. You can visit their website at keephopealive.org.

===========================================

## Patients – where to find a physician in your area

If you are considering trying ozone, your best choice is to find a local health care professional trained in bio-oxidative therapies including hyperbaric chambers, ozone autohemotherapy and hydrogen peroxide by contacting the American College for Advancement in Medicine (**www.acamnet.org**) or by calling them at 800-532-3688. They keep an updated list of health care professionals trained in a wide range of progressive medical treatment including EDTA chelation – (an alternative to bypass surgery to open partially blocked arteries and reverse athereosclerosis), environmental illness, nutrition, holistic medicine and much more.

## H2O2 Resources

Consumers - check with your local health food store or health care professional. Doctors – check under chemical suppliers in your local phone directory.
If not locally available write to –
Sprout Master Ontario Canada 705-322-2222 sproutmaster.com
Al Myers, PO Box 2508, Clovis, CA 93613 (offer 7% food grade H2O2 solution)
Family Health News, 9845 NE $2^{nd}$ Ave, Miami Shores, FL 33138

---

*****Hydrozone and Glycozone**, by Charles Marchand, Chemist. First published 1904. Reprinted 1989. **Hydrogen Peroxide - Medical Miracle**, by Dr. William C. Douglass M.D. For a list of these and all other available books on oxidative therapies, write to ECHO, PO Box 126, Delano, MN 55328 or do a search on the internet at amazon.com or other web sites that sell books.

---

*Hydrogen Peroxide & Ozone* (you are reading it) - Copies of this booklet are available from Nutri Books 303-778-8383 or from the publisher, Vital Health Publications - 414-329-0648. Use this number to also contact the author of this book.

## Procedures for treating accidental ingestion of 35% H2O2

The danger from consuming too much hydrogen peroxide too fast is the development of a gas embolism in the blood that could cause a stroke or even kill you. That is why I have written several warnings in this book particularly about the dangers of the home use of 35% H2O2 – to never store hydrogen peroxide in any bottle other than a brown or black bottle (never a clear bottle). Also to limit the amount to 2 to 4 ounces per bottle and include a built in dropper dispenser. Ffinally - NEVER STORE HYDROGEN PEROXIDE OR ANY STRENGTH IN A REFRIGERATOR WHERE IT COULD BE MISTAKEN FOR SOMETHING EDIBLE.

If accidental ingestion occurs in children (over 1 teaspoon or more) or adults (1 tablespoon or more) of 35% H2O2, take the following steps immediately.

**1. Drink one pint of fruit juice or water** and follow with a second pint if possible. This slows down the rate of absorption of H2O2 from the stomach.

**2. Take person to hospital and ask to have the fluid pumped out of the stomach** and especially if a child is involved.

**3. If step 2 is not implemented within 10 minutes after ingestion, do any of the following** to slow down the absorption of the H2O2 from the stomach – eat as many **dry crackers** as the patient can eat and as much fruit juice or water as the person can immediately drink. If Metamucil or other fiber mix is available, add that to the drink to slow absorption. Keep feet straight up and elevated above the head to help keep oxygen bubbles out of head for next 8 hours and take patient to the nearest Emergency Room. Take these instructions along. **Note: reports on Medlline (NLM) that a hyperbaric chamber prevented gas embolism in a patient that accidentally drank 35% H2O2.**

But it doesn't matter what the "ologists" think, because there's something much more sinister than shifting tectonic plates happening here. I believe, at the center of the Earth, there are hundreds, maybe thousands, of Rock People . . . HAVING A PARTY!

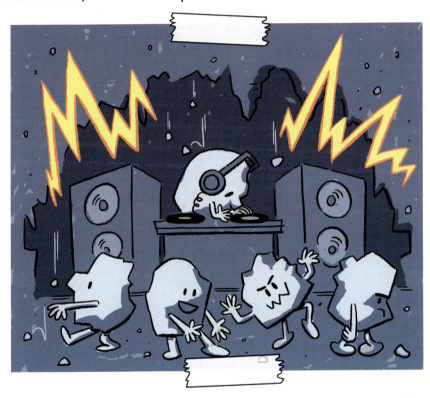

Like most parties, I wasn't invited. Probably because I don't have pebbles for blood. The Rock People must've been celebrating something big, because I could feel that music booming all the way up on the surface. I fear it was a celebration of the commencement of their CONQUEST OF EARTH. We have little time left, people. We must mobilize! Or at least throw a bigger party to show that WE'RE NOT AFRAID!

# WEIRDILOGUE/THE END, QUESTION MARK?

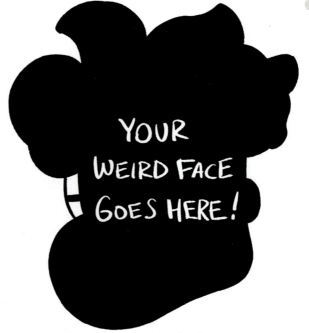

Well, you've reached the end of the book, and proven yourself worthy of handling the TRUTH. But this is not the end of my investigations – not by a long shot! There are new mysteries happening every day, and not just in Beach City! My town may be the weirdest, but I encourage you to start your own investigations. I'm sure if you look hard enough, you'll discover weird stuff in your own city or town . . . or DIMENSION?! Consider yourself deputized as an official WEIRDO!

Normal is boring! Keep Beach City Weird and Keep Your Town Weird!!!